The 30-Day Home Workout Plan

The Easy Way to Keep in Shape at Home and Gain Strength

By: BIRDIE CARA WRIGHT

TABLE OF CONTENTS

INTRODUCTION

As a certain politician likes to say "the debate is settled" when it comes to the total benefits of a healthy, consistent fitness regimen. The body of research on the life- extending (or life-saving, in some instances) attributes of daily exercise is overwhelming, so, for this post, we will dispense with listing all of the physiological and psychological benefits that accrue to those who faithfully pursue optimal fitness. Anyone who isn't fully versed on the advantages of fitness is either in denial or has willfully accepted the consequences of a sedentary lifestyle and they're probably not reading this post anyway.

Granted, beginning and maintaining a daily fitness regimen is challenging, however, it's no more challenging than developing any other habit - which is an acquired pattern of behavior that occurs automatically, without thought. Once it becomes a habit, we tend to break through walls for a "fix" - think golf, coffee, cigarettes, chocolate, or any other habit, good or bad, that controls your life. Soon, it becomes an addiction, which your mind and your body will crave to the point of punishing you with illness or depression when it is deprived.

THE BEAUTY OF AT-HOME WORKOUTS

You probably know of relatives or friends who have gotten awesome results by hitting the local gym and hiring a personal trainer. Yes, it's the classic weight loss story. Still, for those who are not enthusiastic about making the commute to the gym, or are too insecure to go to the gym, going to the gym may sound like a one-way ticket to diet failure.

Going to the gym doesn't have to have to be the only solution. In order to achieve sustainable weight loss you may need to consider doing at-home workouts. Sometimes, the best option is to have an at-home workout that is guided by an at-home personal training service or by developing your own workout. That is the main way to achieve sustainable weight loss. Working out whether at-home or at the gym needs to be convenient. The Holy Grail of weight loss is sustainability.

The benefits to having an at-home workout are many not to mention it is sustainable. For those who are looking for the utmost convenience without all the problems that going to a gym may have, an at-home workout plan may be the fitness solution that they need. It requires no driving time, no dealing with other people, and you can work out whenever you want. Since you can work out whenever and wherever you want with an at-home workout schedule, it allows people who need a high level of flexibility to get in shape causing it to be sustainable. The beauty is that it's convenient and science has even shown that it can be just as effective as weight training at the gym!

An at-home workout can be just as effective as a workout that you would have at the gym - even if you don't have the same equipment that you would find at a gym. This is because it is not the equipment that makes an effective workout it's the workout intensity and design. What makes an effective workout is the right routine that targets the right muscle groups and allows your body to burn fat throughout your body and even after the workout is over. Functional strength training via body weight training requires no specialized equipment, can be done anywhere, and totally works your entire body! A good workout schedule will also raise you to your optimal fitness level, improve your metabolism, and also improve your general wellbeing. Since every individual is a little different, you should look for a personalized at-home workout that will help you lose weight, tone up, get into shape, and most importantly is sustainable.

It is well known that most personal fitness routines that are at-home in nature tend to be cheaper than a gym membership, especially if you take the services of a personal trainer along with the membership. Either way both are equally as effective at helping you get in shape. Getting you in shape at-home or at the gym in a sustainable fashion is the main goal of any fitness program no matter the cost. If you are looking for a workout that will get you in shape, improve your general health, and is convenient, it's time to start taking a look at our at-home workouts. Stop by and see what we offer when it comes to bodyweight exercises. You will be surprised at how great you will feel and how your quality of life can improve tremendously.

BENEFITS OF WORKING OUT AT HOME

Whether you need to burn more calories or boost your stamina, you know you don't have to go to the gym to achieve your goals. In fact, you can easily exercise in the comfort of your own home. There are many reasons why you might want to give up on that gym membership and start experiencing the benefits of working out at home...

No Distractions

Don't you ever get the feeling that some people go to the gym just to make new friends instead of working out? Don't get me wrong, there's nothing wrong with that... But if your main goal is to get in shape, then you might want to avoid being distracted by others. If you work out at home, you'll be able to focus and get things done.

No Stress

You're at the gym. You want to try a new workout but you get the feeling that everyone is watching you. Maybe they'll make fun of you.

Some people will tell you it's all in your head. Even if everyone else is focused on their own workout, you can't help it. You still think they're watching you...

At home, you can avoid all the stress in the world. Get rid of the paranoia. Even if you really want to try that new workout, no one is there to judge you. No one will give you some advice you never asked for.

Freedom

Enjoy your workout whenever you want – wherever you want. Feel like working out on a treadmill at midnight? Since your home gym is open 24/7 all you have to do is start right away… You're in control: set up your own rules and exercise at your own pace while listening to your favorite music to help you get in the mood.

Save Time

Think about all the things you need to do when you go to the gym:

- Wake up early
- Get dressed
- Spend more time in your car
- Change into your workout clothes
- Chat with other people
- Do the actual workout
- Get in line to use the equipment you want

If you have your own gym, you'll be saving some time. The only thing you'll have to think about is the actual workout.

Save Money

Not only a gym membership will cost you money, but you're likely to spend some of it on gas too. If you work out at home, you'll avoid both problems. You'll definitely save some money in the long run if you purchase the right equipment for you.

THE WORKOUT ROUTINES OF TODAY

If you find yourself in the ever-growing category of those that are obsessed with hitting specific goals in regards to their health and weight-loss there are a few new exciting options available today. It seems the workout routines of the past which were antiquated and boring have been revamped to deliver routines that are motivating them to bring real results.

The days when you had to drop to the floor to do hundreds of situps or become extremely exhausted doing what seemed to be thousands of jumping jacks are gone. Not to mention there's no forgetting that ridiculously repetitive running in place. The type of exercises just mentioned above as being inefficient are just plain boring, in fact, mustering up some motivation to do them on a daily basis can be harder than actually doing the exercises themselves. As those exercise routines get tossed out the window so do the goals you set in regards to your weight and health.

The workout routines of today consist of any of the following mentioned programs from going to your local gym or fitness center, to purchasing equipment of your own that you can use in home, to even buying in home DVD-based workout programs. Not to mention this is the Internet age and there are all kinds of custom programs and plans online that can be tailored to meet your needs. These plans can vary depending on your age, current health, and the results that you're looking to get from the program.

Anyone just starting out would begin with simple workout routines that incorporate low impact repetitions this being the best way to go. Your workouts should never leave you out of breath or without the wish to keep on going, nor injure any particular muscle group. A simple beginning workout routine would include exercises that are well known, for instance crunches that focus on the midsection. This particular workout would perhaps for the beginner be performed in sets of 3 to 5 with several breaks in between working up to a completion of 25 reps. From this point the new exerciser can move on to other exercises that work other areas of the body for instance the biceps.

Starting with dumbbells for your biceps you'd want to get into a habit of performing 3 sets of reps with each set consisting of no more than 12 reps per arm. As your body becomes accustomed to the weight at that time it would be good to increase the weight of your dumbbells for added resistance. A crucial point to keep in mind is that as you increase your weight avoid increasing it dramatically as this can lead to an overtaxing of your muscles.

There are also levels of exercise routines for intermediate and advanced individuals. These are usually reserved for those who wish to maintain results already achieved or to speed up a weight loss program. The intermediate and advanced program consists of the same exercises previously mentioned but contain more variation and more aggressive repetitions. For example, the abdominal curls are now added to "tuck crunches", with all exercises being done for up to twenty-five reps. Of course, don't forget to rest between sets!

Although ab exercises have been focused on in this section you also are given varying levels of a hamstring, forearm, legs, back, shoulders and cardio routines that are in place to get those areas of your body in shape. Making a fitness accessory purchase can also go a long way to increase the results you get from your routine. As an example consider a resistance band which can be used to help tone almost every part of your body. As an inexpensive accessory the ban can be used when you're lying down, standing, or squatting against a wall. The band is best used when it's placed underneath your feet and you pull on the handles upwards or outwards feeling the resistance in your arms, shoulders, back and chest.

Another position where the bands can be handy would be when you're in a reclining position and the bands are under your feet while you pull towards your body for tension engaging all kinds of upper and lower body muscles. The resistance band is probably one of the best accessories any beginner can buy. In addition to resistance bands a few other accessories that should be added to any workout routine would be dumbbells of varying weights, wrist or ankle weights as well as a heart rate monitor.

Of course all these suggestions about a great working exercise routine would completely null and void that routine if it did not come with the best possible nutritional eating plan. In accordance with any exercise plan must be a healthy diet plan to back it up. When someone eats right and nutritiously while on a workout or fitness plan they are improving the odds dramatically that their metabolism will work properly and that their body as a whole will function and perform better. Proper nutrition also goes a great distance in helping out your immune system, your brains alertness and response time as well as your skin.

When an adequate diet and proper nutrition is avoided your body will respond by disappointing you rendering all of your exercise energies useless. What's even more is that once you begin to see the results coming from your better eating habits you will have more motivation to increase the amount of time you exercise and give it your all.

The best diet for a workout routine or actually anyone alive today hands down would be a diet made up of foods that are rich in vitamins, fats, fiber, carbohydrates, minerals and protein. Try not to forget about water either - when water is readily available it helps your body to stay hydrated due to the fact that regular exercise saps your body of its essential moisture. When considering the best diet for you just think back to the food pyramid you were taught in school.

Your teachers had the right idea when they stressed the importance of getting in at least five servings of nutritious and healthy fruits and vegetables per day.

Today the reasons for being healthy and staying fit are well-known by most people. The benefits you get from this type of lifestyle allow you to not just look better but also feel better. When proper workout routines are incorporated into your lifestyle you will immediately feel the benefits and enjoy a longer more satisfying life as well.

EASY AT HOME EXERCISES

Exercise at Home - No Equipment, No Problem!

You have a million things to do and spending 2 hours at the gym just isn't one of them. Sometimes there just isn't enough hours in a day. If you exercise at home you cut out all that driving time and it seems more manageable. Having said that, don't think you're off the the hook. We can still get your heart rate up, boost your metabolism, and get results all in the comfort of you own home.

The secret to getting the most out of your workout at home, and in the gym, is performing your workout in the form of a circuit. By moving from one strength training exercise to the next you will get you heart rate up and knock out strength training and cardio in a matter of 30 minutes and leave your metabolism elevated for hours...all without e?uipment!

Here's the plan.You are going to perform five exercises with no rest in between. If you are just getting started allow yourself to rest 15-20 seconds in between each move and work your way up to not resting at all. At the completion of all five exercise you will rest for 1-2 minutes. Then, move on to the next five exercises and perform them in the same fashion. Repeat the two groups of exercises 1-2 more times.

Group 1

1. Push-ups: 15 reps

- Lie face down with legs extended out behind you and feet together
- Place your hands slightly wider than shoulders width apart, palms down, elbows at a 90 degree angle
- Wide Push-up Option:

- Start with hands about 3 inches wider that the regular push-up
- Straighten arms, keeping abs tight and lift up on your toes (or knees for a modified version)so your body is flat like a table...get that butt out of the air!
- Keeping your body straight, lower body to the ground by bending your elbows until your upper arms are parallel with the floor
- Return to the start position by pushing yourself back up

Important:

- Keep your spine in line by keeping your eyes focused on the floor and your abs tight...don't let your body sag on the way up. Also, exhale on the way up and inhale on the way down.Important: Get your butt out of the air! And don't let your body sag! Keep your back straight, your spine in line and just hold the position.

2. Squats: 25 reps

- Stand with feet about shoulder width apart, weight on heels, abs pulled in and good posture
- Using weight...hold dumbbell with both hands directly in front of your body
- Lower yourself down and back by bending your knees. Stick your butt out and keep a straight back
- Lower yourself down until your upper thigh is parallel to the ground (almost as if you are about to sit on a chair)
- Dumbbell hangs straight down in between legs
- Exhale Return to the start position by straightening your legs
- At the top, squeeze your butt cheeks together like you are picking up a $100 bill
- Turn them into jump squats for more of a challenge

Important:

- Never let your knees extend past your toes. Keep a straight back. Don't lean forward (shoulders back) and don't let heals lose contact with the ground.

3. Abdominal Planks: 45-60 seconds

- Start in push-up position: back straight, legs directly behind you, up on your toes,hands directly under shoulders and arms straight
- you can start out on your knees and work up to being on your toes
- You are balancing your weight on the palms of your hands and the balls of your feet
- Hold this position for as long as you can...start with a goal of 30sec and work up to a minute plus
- Place your hands further out in front for more of a challenge

4. Lunges: 15 on each leg

- Stand with good posture
- Feet together
- Step straight out with one foot about 2 feet
- Lower upper body toward the ground keeping front knee behind toe and shin perpendicular to ground
- Push back up with front leg and return to start position with a controlled movement
- Switch and repeat
- Important:
- Knee should not touch ground. When knee extends out passed the toes this causes unnecessary stress on knee. Also, keep a good posture...try not to lean forward

5. Jumping Jacks: 60 seconds

- You know the drill

Group 2

1. Pelvic Thrusts: 15 on each leg

- Lie on your back with your heels on a bench or chair...your legs should make a 90 degree angle
- With your arms relaxed at your side, raise the left leg up so it is pointed toward the sky...keep foot flexed (don't point your toe)
- Pressing the right heel into the bench or chair, drive your left heel straight up toward the sky by lifting your hips
- Pause and slowly lower your body down until it almost touches the floor...repeat for instructed number of reps and switch legs

Important:

- Remember to breathe. Exhale as you drive your leg toward the sky and inhale on the way down.

2. Tricep Dips:15 reps

- Position yourself with your butt just off the edge of bench or chair with hands next to your hips, fingers curled under chair, knuckles facing forward
- Feet are out in front of you at a 90 degree angle (more advanced - legs out straight, motivated- heels on another chair or stability ball)
- Lower your body toward the ground by bending at the elbows

* Go as far as you can or until your arms are at a 90 degree angle
* Return to the start position by straightening your arms
* Inhale on the way down, and exhale on the way up

Important:

* Don't let your elbows flare out. Don't let your chest collapse as you lower down. Don't perform this exercise if you have a shoulder injury or wrist pain

3. Chair Sits 20 seconds, rest for 5 seconds, back down for 20 more seconds

* Stand with your feet together, good posture, weight on your heels
* Bend your knees and lower your butt to the ground until your upper leg is almost parallel to the ground...don't let your knees get over your toes
* Bend forward slightly at the waist
* Keeping your arms straight, raise your arms up to the sky until they are right by your ears
* Jump your feet up toward your hands and land so you are in the squat position
* Now jump straight up in the air, getting your feet off the ground and reaching for the sky
* Land in the squat position, place your hands back on the floor and jump your feet back to the push-up position

Important:

* Keep your knees behind your toes and weight on your heels. Don't let those arms drop...we don't want your shoulders to miss out on the fun!

4. Superman: 15 reps and hold for 15 seconds after last rep

- Lie face down with legs straight out behind you and arms straight out in front of you...like Superman
- Lift you arms, chest and legs off the floor...squeeze your butt cheeks and hold for a beat!
- Return to the start position, but don't let your feet and hands touch the ground. They should hover a couple of inches above the ground.

Important:

- Nice, slow controlled movement

5. Mt. Climbers: 60 seconds

- Start in the plank/push-up position with your body in a straight line, hands directly under your shoulders
- Jump your left foot forward driving your knee up toward your chest (left foot stays off the ground)
- Your right foot stays out behind you in the start position
- Very quickly, return your left foot to the start position and simultaneously, repeat the same move with the right foot
- Repeat at a rapid pace for the instructed amount of time

USER FRIENDLY HABITS FOR SUCCESSFUL HOME GYM TRAINING

Are you dissatisfied with your current training program? Are you not achieving the results you had hoped for when you started training? If you are you stuck on a fitness plateau and are in need of some tips on how to start seeing progress then keep reading.

I am sure you want to see results from your training program (why would you do it if you didn't want to see results, right?). You can start seeing measurable results again and break through those training plateaus by incorporating one or more of the following success habits for successful home gym training. In my ten+ years involved in the fitness industry and helping hundreds of people achieve their fitness goals, I have found these habits very valuable tools when it comes to seeing results from your training. I recommend using the ones that work for you and breaking through that training plateau!

Fitness Success Habits:

Set Clear Goals

Unfortunately a lot of people head to the gym without clearly identifying what it is exactly that they want to achieve. I suggest you nail down a specific goal to train for. I have found that when my clients really nail down a purpose to train for they always get better results. I find it interesting that when people focus on training for a special event they usually see better body composition results even though they weren't focusing on that. I recommend picking a road race a few weeks out, a list of mountains to hike, a special date to look your best at, or a special competition to get ready for.

Select "Money" Exercises

Simply put, some exercises deliver a lot more benefit than others. Multi-joint, compound exercises like snatches, cleans, squats, deadlifts, lunges, step-ups, bench presses, chest presses, seated rows, bentover rows, standing overhead presses, lat. pulldowns, pull-ups and chin-ups should make up the core of your exercise selection. No matter what your goals are you will get far better results by making the exercises listed above the core of your training program.

Keep a Training Log

"But, I don't need a training log, I can remember what I have done before in my head." I hear this one all the time, usually from the same people who are not seeing any results from their efforts. Listen. If you want to see progress from your training, don't leave things up to guess work. Remove all doubt and start tracking things. Track your progress via measurements such as body fat percentage, girth measurements, and body weight. Your training log can help you learn from your prior mistakes and help you achieve the results you are looking for at a faster rate.

Have a Plan

Now that you have a compelling goal to train for you need a plan. I hang out in gyms a lot and most of the time I see people wandering around the gym with no plan at all. If people do have a plan that they are following, often times the plan is not appropriate for that individual. The best advice I can find is to get an individualized plan suited to the goals you have laid out. See habit number 10 below to learn more about getting the right plan for you.

Use Progressive Overload

"If you do what you have always done, you will get what you have always gotten." You need to progress in order to make your body change. This is a key habit that should be followed when it comes to training the human body. In order to see the physical changes you are looking for, you want to focus on improving from workout to workout. You can perform one or more reps than last time, lift a slightly heavier weight, and do the same amount of work in less time. The key is to challenge the body by progressively and systematically overloading the body in an intelligent manner.

Utilize Planned Variety

On average, the typical individual will adapt to an exercise program in 3-6 weeks. If you have been following a specific routine and you are not seeing results, then it is probably time to start mixing things up. You can change all kinds of things to get some needed variety in your program. You can change the overall format (switch to circuit training, supersets, etc.), change the number of sets, change the number of reps per set, change the rest periods between sets, change the exercises you are using for a given muscle group, change the grip or hand position, and you can even change the speed of movement for the exercises. The options are almost unlimited so don't bore your muscles with the same old exercises with the same old 3 sets of 10 repetitions. Variety is the spice of life and a key factor in seeing continued progress.

Track What You Eat

Some experts say that 75-80% of your overall results are totally due to your nutrition. This may be surprising to you but you can gain muscle or lose fat on the exact same program. Your nutritional intake will totally dictate your results so if you really want to make some progress it can be a good idea to periodically track what you eat so that you can make sure that you are eating in a manner supportive to your goals.

Periodically Evaluate Your Progress or Lack Thereof

No program works forever and no matter how effective a given program was you should mix things up when you are no longer seeing results from your efforts. The only way to judge the effectiveness of a training program is by the results it is producing or not producing. Some experts recommend checking your progress every 1-3 weeks to see if you are improving in the areas you want to. If you are not seeing improvements then that should be a mental note for you to make some changes. If you are seeing results, keep training until that program no longer delivers.

Find a Great Training Partner

A great training habit that has the potential to improve your fitness results is to find a dedicated training partner. Choose carefully. You want someone who will challenge you, someone positive, someone to keep you on track, and someone who will help improve your training. You don't want someone who is unreliable, negative, and lazy. Choose wisely and this training habit could mean renewed progress!

Find Coaches and Mentors

Coaches and Mentors can help save you lots of frustration. Coaches and Mentors have been there before and help you achieve better results at a faster rate. They know little tricks to help you get back on track towards the results you want, so do yourself a favor and invest in yourself by learning from these experienced teachers.

HOW TO EXERCISE AT HOME

Although many people plan to get fit every year, very few do. One of the primary reasons people don't improve their fitness is that they think they need to go to the gym to get in shape. Going to the gym is great if you can afford it and have the time to go regularly, but you can get in better shape without ever setting foot inside a gym. Don't let your inability to join a gym stop you from achieving the fitness level you deserve. Start working out in your own home at your own pace and watch your body change from flabby to fit in accordance with your dreams.

Every workout should begin with an exercise for your heart. Any kind of exercise that gets your heart pumping a little faster is good for you. It not only makes your heart and lungs stronger, but also helps energize you and promotes a positive mood. If you're prone to depression, exercise of this nature is an important part of your daily routine; even if you don't suffer from depression, you are missing out on benefits if you don't start with a cardio workout.

You can do just about any exercise you enjoy, as long as it gets your heart pumping. If you have exercise equipment in your home such as a stationary bike or a treadmill, that's ideal for cardio workouts. You can also use exercise DVDs or search for exercise videos on YouTube.

Don't overdo your cardio workout. Start small and then gradually build the intensity or the time you spend exercising. Eventually, you want to do 20 minutes a day of moderate cardio exercise five days a week.

After you finish your cardio routine, you might want to do some additional exercise to tone your muscles. Most gyms have weight machines to help you build muscles and tone the muscles you already have, but if you're at home you may not have access to weights.

Instead, you can do some traditional exercises similar to the ones that you probably did in gym class when you were a child. Incorporate exercises such as push-ups and pull-ups into your daily exercise routine. After you've finished these exercises, follow them up with jumping jacks and squats. This routine allows you to build both upper and lower body muscles.

After you've finished working out, it's important to stretch. Working out puts extra pressure on your muscles because you use them in ways you may not be used to. After working out, your muscles are warm and loose; when they cool down they may suddenly contract and tear. This causes you to feel sore. If you stretch after working out, it loosens the muscles further. This makes it less likely that you will injure your muscles and feel sore following a workout.

Going to the gym sometimes motivates people to exercise, but it isn't really necessary. You may find it easier to exercise in your own home. If you make it part of your daily routine to turn on that exercise DVD or get on the exercise bike when you get up, soon you'll find yourself losing weight, building muscle and having fun--all without leaving your house.

THE BEST HOME GYMS FOR YOUR WORKOUTS

Home fitness gyms are quite popular for people who want the benefits of a good workout without having to leave home to get it. The best home gyms on the market are durable, reliable, constructed with quality parts and materials, and most importantly, meet your specific fitness and workout needs.

Three Types of Home Gyms

There are three basic types of home gym:

- Machine
- Free weight
- Plate loaded machine

Each type comes with its own advantages and disadvantages, and each is suited to different workout needs and styles. Determining the best home gyms for your consideration requires some research and information gathering to narrow the list to a few you can try out in person.

Let's take a look at each of these in turn.

About Machine Home Gyms

Machine home gyms are constructed of a single steel frame. Attached to this frame are different types of training equipment that work different parts of the body with different motions and exercises.

Machine home gyms generally fall into three categories:

Traditional

This is the most common type of machine home gym. It contains multiple stations and functions, such as a lat pull down, leg extension and leg curl, press, and bench. Most also have an adjustable weight stack and may also have a low row station, too.

Power rod

This category uses flexible rods to create resistance and weight load during your workout. The rods are of varying stiffness and thus create various levels of resistance. The most well known power rod home gym is the Bowflex brand.

Gravity resistance

This category of machine home gyms is typically lightweight, portable, and of somewhat questionable quality. The machine has a metal frame that is adjustable, and a gliding bench or board that holds your body during exercises. The weight of your body creates the resistance, as you pull on cables to glide yourself up and down various inclines and in various positions.

About Free Weight Home Gyms

A free weight home gym consists of several separate pieces of equipment that are not attached together in any way. The pieces are used in different combinations and different frequencies to achieve training goals. Weights are added, dropped or adjusted by hand, using whichever bar you have selected for a particular exercise.

Free weight home gyms generally fall into three categories:

Traditional

This is the most common category and considered by many to be the best home gyms for multi-purpose workouts. The specific components may vary, but usually include at least one barbell, two dumbbells, a variety of weight plates, a bench and rack, and collars to prevent weight plates from falling.

Power rack

This category is generally for home gyms that focus on heavy exercises. The power rack itself is free standing and holds the barbell. The user adjusts the height of the rack so that he or she squats slightly to place the barbell across the top of the back, then stands up straight and moves back to commence the exercise. When the exercise is complete, the user simply moves forward again and places the barbell back in the rack.

Power cage

This category of eＱuipment is used in much the same manner as a power rack, but with a slight difference. The power cage has rectangular sides for holding the barbell, which means the user cannot move as far forward or backward as they can with power rack eＱuipment.

About Plate Loaded Machine Home Gyms

A plate loaded machine home gym combines elements of both a free weight home gym and a standard machine home gym. It may have several stations and functions like a machine home gym, but instead of having a standard weight stack it requires you to add and subtract weight by hand, just like with a free weight home gym.

There are three common categories of plate loaded machine home gyms:

Machine without weight stacks

This category is for equipment that is essentially a standard machine home gym with multiple stations, but with the exception that weights are loaded manually.

Smith machine

This category is a machine-form of a power rack or a power cage. Instead of the user moving backward to perform the actual exercises, a smith machine limits the motion to straight up and down without any forward or backward movement.

Combination Smith machine

This category combines the elements of a standard smith machine with some of the things found on a machine gym, such as a lat pull down or other similar function.

Which Gym is Best For You?

The best home gyms are those that have the features and functions that match your personal fitness goals and meet other specific requirement.

For example, if your goal is to build gigantic muscles then you should consider a smith machine that allows you to do squats, dead lifts, and perform both with a great deal of weight. If your goals are more modest, though, then a standard machine home gym should be sufficient. You might even prefer a gravity resistance home gym if you are more interested in overall body toning rather than building up muscle bulk.

Of course, cost is a big consideration, and as with most other types of fitness equipment, you will tend to get a level of quality that is in line with the amount of money that you spend. Many people opt for a short term membership at a gym or fitness club so that they can try several types of machines to see which ones they like best.

Still not sure which is right for you? Think about buying an inexpensive home gym of whatever type you like the best so you can try it out without making a huge financial commitment. If you are ready to take the plunge and invest in a high quality, serious fitness home gym, though, expect to spend at least $500 and more likely around $1,000 or more.

Before making any purchase, it is critical that you measure the space where you plan to put your home gym so you know exactly how big your home gym should be. Remember to allow enough space around the perimeter of the home gym so that you can easily move around and access the equipment.

POWERFUL WAYS TO MOTIVATE YOURSELF TO WORKOUT

More than likely, because of this Coronavirus lockdown, your motivation to workout at home is less than your motivation to workout in the gym. At home you get distracted, others interrupt you, a program on TV takes away your attention. And there are many other commotions that get in the way.

So what do you do?

How do you avoid those disruptions? How can you motivate yourself to workout regularly and correctly?

The key question to ask yourself is, How badly do you want to achieve your health and fitness goal?

How to motivate yourself to workout is simple. Answer that question. Think about it with focused intensity. See the goal that you want to achieve in your mind, and reiterate your goal and, more importantly, reiterate the reason why you want to achieve that goal.

What's the WHY you want to be fit and healthy.

What do you want to be fit and healthy for?

The WHY possesses all the power to go after your goal until it is achieved - even if you are working out from home in this lockdown situation.

How much you want your goal determines the strength of your motivation.

It is that strength that will steadfastly motivate and drive you to fulfil your goal irrespective of any challenges, setbacks, oppositions, confrontations, distractions, interruptions, diversions, or anything else.

How to stay motivated will not be an issue anymore!

I recall a friend who set himself a goal that he felt extremely excited about. He talked for days on end about that goal; what it meant to him and how he really wanted to achieve it within six months at the most.

A couple of months later, my friend Bill, took me aside. I could see he was feeling miserable and despondent. He went on to tell me how disappointed he was that his goal had not materialised.

"Goal! What Goal?" was my honest answer. I had forgotten all about it. It was not what Bill wanted to hear.

"You know, my goal to get a toned, sculptured beach body," Bill reminded me, with a deep sense of defeat and frustration echoing from his voice.

"Oh that. I thought you were kidding. We all figured you changed your mind since we don't see you going to the gym anymore," I replied, perhaps a little sarcastically.

So, what happened here? What happened to Bill's drive? Where's his motivation?

In the beginning, Bill was excited about his new goal of getting a firm and toned beach body as he put it. He was full of motivation and determination to achieve that goal. "I will get it no matter what," where his last words to me. Hmmm.

He consistently went to the gym four to five days a week. He took his protein shakes, his supplements, and always asked personal trainers' questions about his training schedule and routine.

He was pleased with his progress.

By the third month, though, he started to go to the gym twice a week, and half-way through that third month it trickled to once a week.

His dilemma was he couldn't understand why his motivation to go to the gum and workout had dwindled to once a week half-way through the third month.

"At the beginning, I was so full of enthusiasm and motivation. I felt nothing could stop me," he explained, feeling ever so confused.

So what went wrong? Where did his incredible and unstoppable motivation go?

After careful examination, it came to light that Bill had lost his burst of motivation because he was not really passionate about being toned.

He really didn't care too much about having that beach body. In fact, he used to laugh at the beach-bodied people whenever he spotted one on holiday.

Interesting point, huh? See where this is going?

His goal was merely a passing 'wish'.

In other words, he did not want to be toned badly enough. If he did, if he felt passionate, he would have continued his workout routine no matter what challenges he faced.

Bill was torn between two thoughts.

The first said, "Yeah, I'd like to have a toned beach body." But his conflicting second thought argued, "Sure, but you could get along in life without it. You laugh at people who have a perfectly toned beach body, now you want one? Come on!"

And who won?

His conflicting thought had the upper hand.

You see, Bill would have 'liked' the toned body, but he did not turn that wish into a solid goal.

The toned body idea remained just that, an idea or a wish. As such, his once powerful motivation had weakened until it was there no more.

If he had turned it into a goal, a solid goal, he would have sought after it. He would have been motivated to pursue that goal irrespective of how tired or how busy he was.

After all, it was his goal. And goals are meant to be achieved.

Passion ignites the drive from deep within to maintain the motivation to reach all sorts of goals.

Passion provides the fuel to keep you in a highly motivated state of mind.

Once you find out what you are passionate about, once you find out the WHY you want to be healthy and fit for, how to motivate yourself to workout will become a simple matter of getting up and getting started no matter what.

Your motivation to remain persistent regardless of any setbacks and obstacles will be unstoppably strong.

Now, in this lockdown situation we are all facing, I have included below powerful ways you can make use of to motivate yourself to workout - in time, your motivation will increase in momentum regardless of any distractions or interruptions.

Motivation fuels you to take consistent daily action to achieve and live your goal.

The powerful ways on how to stay motivated are listed below. All you have to do is alter your strategy:

Plan your health and fitness goal once again

Now that you are in lockdown mode, simply having a goal will not mean you can achieve it. Your mind is too focused on this interruption of you going to the gym. By being frustrated and continually asking yourself, "How can I stay motivated with all these interruptions around me? How can I stay motivated without being surrounded by others who are also working out?" and an array of other similar questions, you will inevitably head towards the wrong direction.

As we saw with Bill, you need to have a clear and concise goal with no conflicts.

Simply wishing to have a certain kind of body won't help.

Simply wishing to lose weight won't help.

Simply wishing to jog the marathon won't help.

Working out has so much more to do with an emotion of achieving complete and all round fitness.

That's a great goal to strive for; at least for now while you're working out at home and not in the gym.

So what workout routine plan can you follow at home? Jumping Jacks, Planks, Tricep Dips using a stable chair? Think about it and come up with a plan. It need not be written in stone; adjust it as time goes by until you finally come up with a plan you'll be happy about.

You may face 'at-home-distractions'. Arrange with the people surrounding you a time of no interruptions while you workout. Ask them to respect your workout time.

Focus on the emotion of working out, and not on just working out

A powerful way to stay motivated to workout is by focusing on the emotion and happiness that working out will bring.

Endure the discomfort of working out at home by seeing the end result; by remembering the WHY you are working out for in the first place.

And an even more powerful emotion booster is to look into the mirror after the workout.

See and feel how great you look. This is a great motivation booster.

Reward yourself

When you used to workout in the gym, did you reward yourself for having such a great workout? If not, you should've.

Now that you are working out from home, it is even more important to reward yourself after each and every workout.

Come up with a list of rewards.

Pamper yourself.

Stick to the plan that works for you

As we mentioned in step one, planning is important. Now, sticking to the final plan is crucial to your fitness success.

If your motivation to workout has dwindled, and it may at times, this is where discipline and your big WHY kick in.

Allow discipline to motivate yourself to workout.

Allow the big WHY to be your powerful 'chatter on your shoulder'; that urges you to stay motivated. This 'chatter on your shoulder' guides you on how to stay motivated throughout your workout.

And throughout the lockdown.

Quality over quantity

This is key. Just because you are at home and not in a gym doesn't mean that the quality of your workout should suffer.

Do not compromise and settle for less.

Do not jeopardise what you have already gained.

True you may need to adjust your home workout. True how to motivate yourself to workout may be an issue (at first). True the Quality of your workout may take a slight knock.

If that is so, find a way around that to regain as much Quality as you can from each workout session, and perform each session with total determination and dedication.

It's all about quality and not Quantity.

Set yourself workout at home milestones

Chunk your final goal into small achievable milestones. You may do this every week, if you like. If, at the gym, your goal was to do 100 pushups and you find it hard to do that at home for whatever reason, chunk that down to achievable milestones by performing the amount you can do at home and scale up to 100.

Start off with baby steps to see what you can and cannot do and increase it incrementally.

This will certainly keep you motivated.

Get yourself a workout buddy

How to stay motivated consistently may still be a struggle every so often. If that happens to you consider finding a workout buddy; someone who will work out with you, and one who will help you maintain your motivation - and you can encourage and motivate him, too.

What a wonderful win-win exchange.

Music keeps you going

If finding a workout buddy is a challenge for you, or that person cannot be there for you as often as you like (even on Facetime), enlist your other workout buddy: Your music playlist.

For many, listening to music can powerfully motivate them to workout.

Are you one of them?

If not, consider that method.

You may be pleasantly surprised how listening to your favourite music can power you up; where you will be motivated and where you can stay motivated to workout.

And for some, they workout even longer and more intensely as they are powered by the loud beats of songs they love.

A fantastic distraction you will enjoy

As we wrap this up, here's a particular distraction I feel you will like. Perform all or part of your workout while watching your favourite TV program.

This will be a pleasant distraction that will take your mind off the unpleasantness of working out at home and not in the gym.

It could be a great distraction if your cardio routine is 'boring' at home. This distraction will override that boredom, don't you think?

Celebrate!

Make it a point to celebrate your success. You could celebrate every workout completion. You could celebrate reaching every milestone. You could celebrate every week of dedicated working out.

Celebrate that you are actually working out at home in the first place and didn't quit now that the gyms being closed.

Come up with a list of celebratory reasons, and enjoy every celebration.

There you have it. Those were 10 powerful ways to motivate yourself to workout and how to stay motivated during this lockdown.

Let me finish off with a quote from Zig Ziglar: People often say that motivation doesn't last. Well, neither does bathing - that's why we recommend it daily.

AVOID THESE TOP WORKOUT MYTHS

Do you know the health and fitness industry is plagued by an over abundance of workout myths? A myth is a fiction or half truth, especially one that forms part of an ideology. Rob tells Jen about a new fitness program that is suppose to deliver amazing results; Jen tells Ted, and Ted then tells Pam, but only half of what Rob said. Confused? Just image how confusing Rob's "cutting edge" theory has become. And the funny thing is, Rob made this up by telling people they will lose 3 inches from their bellies, and hips by holding their breath for 30 seconds. Rob, without any scientific backing, dreamed this all up.

The sad thing is most people believe what they hear from so-called uninformed myth spreaders. After consulting with thousands of people, I have heard every possible workout myth known to man, and continue to de-bunk myths daily. Listed below are my all time 5 favorite workout myths. Always look for the science and logic behind what people claim. Don't automatically assume it is true unless studies back it, or specific Quantitative results are shown.

After reading my 5 workout myths, you will be able to finally protect your own workout results, and share the fitness truth with others.

Doing crunches, or abdominal work will decrease fat in the stomach area (If you do thousands of crunches, then you will have a flat stomach.)

This is what some infomercials preach. They state you can obtain a flat, beautiful, stomach by using their simple ab machine. All you need to do is exercise 2 minutes per day, and voila!

Please note, dear reader, you can't SPOT REDUCE! By doing a specific exercise for a certain muscle does not make fat suddenly vanish. Fat is lost over time by burning more calories than the body consumes on a regular basis. Fat will then disappear throughout your entire body, and you don't have control of where it comes off. Doing a certain exercise for a specific muscle will only guarantee a stronger, more fit muscle.

The SECRET keys to fat loss are decreasing caloric intake, increasing activity for an extended period of time, and incorporating a workout of strength, cardio, and flexibility.

Lifting heavy weight for 8-12 reps will build big muscles (especially women.) You should lift very light weights and do a lot of reps, 20 +.

This is one that NEVER seems to go away. It keeps coming back to haunt me again, and again, and again. Ladies, doing heavier weights WILL NOT suddenly turn you into the Incredible Hulk. Your objective should be to maintain, or slightly increase your fat burning lean tissue. In order to do this you must increase the intensity of the exercise by elevating weight, number of reps, or decreasing rest time between sets.

If you increase intensity regularly, you will see good results. If you do not, you will get the same results you have been getting. Increase the intensity until you are happy with the progress you have made, and then maintain the same intensity level.

Women, generally, don't have the physiological make-up to develop big muscles unless they use steroids, and train with gut busting intensity. Most men workout a lifetime, and won't build big muscles. Ladies, please don't worry; challenge yourself in the gym.

Here is a valuable free resource to help you stay informed of the health, and fitness trends by letting you know what works, and what doesn't.

For resistance training, you need to do 3 sets of 10-15 reps, 3 exercises per body part, and a frequency of 3 days per week.

Where the heck did 3 come from? 3 X 3 X 3? I think someone, many years ago, decided 3 was a good number to use, and people started to believe in this myth.

How many sets are really needed? According to scientific studies, the exact number of sets needed to stimulate lean tissue development is one, if preformed at 100% momentary muscle failure. A single all out set is the ideal stimulus to trigger lean tissue development. All other sets only hinder the recovery process when lean tissue develops.

Rest- people generally don't get enough rest between workouts. Please be aware that the higher the intensity, the more rest is required between workouts to allow lean tissue development. If you workout (strength train) too soon, before you are fully recovered, you will short circuit your results.

It is better to wait longer between workouts, then to workout not fully recovered.You WON'T lose your muscle tissue if you don't workout for 2 weeks.

Ideal rest times (depending upon intensity) are anywhere from 3 - 10 + days between strength training workouts.

You will need to track your progress to determine when your gains cease. When progress stops, increase your rest time even further.

If your strength keeps increasing during each workout, you are assured of getting optimal rest between sessions.

All I need to do is cardiovascular training to be in shape.

Wrong! Please don't make this mistake! Cardiovascular exercise is only one piece of the workout puzzle. To design an optimal fitness program, incorporate cardiovascular exercise, strength training, and flexibility into an efficient, results producing program.

Cardiovascular exercise will do very little to increase your flexibility, and maintain or increase your lean tissue. If you avoid any of these three components, you are decreasing your results by one third.

As a result of the aging process, on average, 5-7 pounds of muscle is lost each decade, that is, if you don't strength train.

All fitness equipment is good if you use it.

All fitness equipment is not created equal, especially home fitness equipment advertised in infomercials. Some pieces of fitness equipment are not well built, and can cause injury to specific individuals resulting from medical limitations.

CONCLUSION

Just because you are doing a home workout does not mean that it can't be as tough or tougher than people who travel to a gym. Once you know where you are going and how you intend to get there, the rest is up to you. Follow your plan, give it 100% effort, eat right, and you'll be on your way to a fit body.